The Pit and the Pendulum Diet

... because dieting is TORTURE

LaVar Riess

The Pit and the Pendulum Diet

Here an unholy mob of torturers with an insatiable thirst for dieting
Once fed their long frenzy.
Now our sanity is safe, the latest fads destroyed,
And health appears where dreadful starvation once was.
[Quatrain composed for the gates of a market to be erected upon the site of the Dieting Club House at Paris.]

I WAS sick—sick unto death with that long agony; and when the doctor at length finished explaining, and I was permitted to sit, I felt that my senses were leaving me. The sentence—the dread sentence of being "weight challenged"—was the last of the distinct diagnosis which reached my ears. After that, the sound of the intrusive voice seemed merged in one dreamy indeterminate hum. It conveyed to my soul the idea of revulsion—perhaps from its association in fancy with the blur of the magazines I perused while in the waiting room before seeing the doctor. This only for a brief period; for presently I heard no more.

Yet, for a while, I saw; but with how terrible an exaggeration! I saw the full lips of my scantily-robed judges staring back at me from the pages of those magazines as if they were repeating the words, "If I can do it, you can do it." The models appeared to me thin—thinner than the sheet upon which I trace these words—and thin even to exaggeration; thin with the intensity of their expression of ease—of immoveable resolution—of strict commitment to inhuman dieting. I saw that the decrees of what to me was Fate, were still issuing from those lips. I saw them writhe with an accusing expression. I saw them fashion the syllables of my name; and I shuddered because no sound succeeded.

I saw, too, for a few moments of delirious horror, the soft and nearly imperceptible waving of the many dieting posters which draped the walls of the doctor's office. And then my vision fell upon the seven main diet brochures upon the counter: the Anti-Carb Diet; the Counting Calories/Points Diet; the Latest Fad or Magazine

The Pit and the Pendulum Diet

Diet; the Liquid/Fasting/Cleansing/Purging/Reset Diet; the Mediterranean Diet; the expensive Prepackaged/Hire-A-Nutritionist Diet; and the vegetarian/vegan/eat-like-a-rabbit Plant-Based Diet.

At first they wore the aspect of charity, and seemed slender angels who would save me; but then, all at once, there came a most deadly nausea over my spirit, and I felt every fibre in my frame thrill as if I had touched the terminals of a car battery, while the angel forms became meaningless visions of far-distant hope, with thoughts of agony, and I saw that from them there would be no help.

And then there stole into my fancy, like a rich musical note, the thought of what sweet rest there must be once I reach my weight goal. The thought came gently and stealthily, and it seemed long before it attained full appreciation; but just as my spirit came at length properly to feel and entertain it, the figures of the magazine judges vanished, as if magically, from before me; the angel brochures sank into nothingness; their hope went out utterly; the blackness of the thought of unsuccessful dieting supervened; all sensations appeared swallowed up in a mad rushing descent as of the soul into Hades. Then silence, and stillness, night were the universe.

I was dazed and knew not how I had returned home or what I was about; but still will not say that all of consciousness was lost. What of it there remained I will not attempt to define, or even to describe; yet all was not lost. In the deepest slumber—no! In delirium—no! In fainting—no! In drowning my sorrows in a carton of ice cream—no! even in binging all is not lost. Else there is no hope for the would-be dieter. Arousing from the most profound of stupors, we break the gossamer web of some daydream. Yet in the second afterward, (so frail may that web have been) we try to remember not what we have done.

The Pit and the Pendulum Diet

In the return to reality from the haze there are two stages; first, that of the sense of mental or spiritual; secondly, that of the sense of physical, existence. It seems probable that if, upon reaching the bloated feeling of the second stage, we could recall the emotional eating of the first, we should find these impressions forcefully in memories of the gulf beyond. And that gulf is—what? How at least shall we distinguish its shadows from those of self-loathing? But if the impressions of what I have termed the first stage, are not, at will, recalled, yet, after long interval, do they not come unbidden, while we marvel whence they come?

She who has never been in shock for the fear of dieting, is not she who finds strange dieting clinics and wildly thin faces in textured ceilings; is not she who beholds floating in mid-air the sad visions of many who whisper of her girth behind her back; is not she who ponders over the smell of some novel dessert—is not she whose brain grows bewildered with the meaning of some condemning diagnosis which has never before arrested her attention.

Amid frequent and thoughtful endeavors to remember; amid earnest struggles to regather some token of the state of seeming gloom into which my soul had lapsed, there have been moments when I have dreamed of success; there have been brief, very brief periods when I have conjured up remembrances which the lucid reason of a later epoch assures me could have had reference only to that condition of seeming unconsciousness.

These shadows of memory tell, indistinctly, of slender magazine figures that lifted and bore me in silence down—down—still down—till a hideous dizziness oppressed me at the mere idea of descending into a never-ending diet. They tell also of a vague horror at my heart, on account of that heart's unnatural rhythm. Then comes a sense of sudden motionlessness throughout all things; as if those who bore me (a ghastly train!) had outrun, in their descent, the limits of willpower, and paused from the wearisomeness of their toil. After this I call to mind tastelessness and cardboard textures; and then all is madness—the madness of a memory which busies itself among forbidden foods.

Very suddenly there came back to my soul motion and sound—the tumultuous motion of the heart, and, in my ears, the sound of its beating. Then a pause in which all is blank. Then again sound, and motion, and touch—a tingling sensation pervading my frame. Then the mere consciousness of existence, without thought—a condition which lasted long. Then, very suddenly, thought, and shuddering terror, and earnest endeavor to comprehend my true state. Then a strong desire to lapse into insensibility. Then a rushing revival of soul and a successful effort to move. And now a full memory of the diagnosis, of the thin magazine models, of the confusion as to which diet to choose, of the doctor's words, of the sickening feeling in my stomach, of the shock. Then entire forgetfulness of all that followed; of all that a later day and much earnestness of endeavor have enabled me vaguely to recall.

So far, I had not opened my eyes. I felt that I lay upon my back, cut off from the world. I reached out my hand, and it fell heavily upon something smooth and hard. There I suffered it to remain for many minutes, while I strove to imagine where and what I could be. I longed, yet dared not to employ my vision. I dreaded the first glance at objects around me. It was not that I feared to look upon things horrible, but that I grew aghast lest there should be nothing to see. At length, with a wild desperation at heart, I quickly opened my eyes. My worst thoughts, then, were confirmed. I was on the floor of the kitchen and the blackness of nightfall encompassed me.

I struggled for breath. The intensity of the night seemed to oppress and stifle me, not only from the physical darkness, but emotional. The atmosphere was intolerably suffocating. I still lay quietly, and made effort to exercise my reason. I brought to mind the imposing diagnosis, and attempted from that point to deduce my real condition. The sentence of dieting pronounced upon me had happened; and it appeared to me that a very long interval of time had passed since the doctor's visit earlier in the day.

Yet not for a moment did I suppose myself in the Twilight Zone. Such a supposition, notwithstanding what we read in fiction, is altogether inconsistent with reality;—but where and in what state was I? Those caught in denial, I knew, succumbed usually at meetings of Overeaters Anonymous (OA), and one of these had been held on this very night, though I had missed it.

Had I been confined to my mental anguish, to await daily sacrifice until I reached my 'ideal' weight, which would not take place for many months? This I at once saw could not be. The craving to satisfy my hunger had been always in immediate demand. Moreover, my destiny, as well as the destiny of all other dieters, is to attain stone cold resolve that there is a light at the end of the tunnel.

A fearful idea now suddenly drove the blood in torrents upon my heart as I perused once more the seven diet brochures, and for a brief period, I once more relapsed into insensibility. Upon recovering, I at once started to my feet, trembling convulsively in every fibre. I thrust my arms wildly above and around me in all directions in exasperation. I felt nothing; yet dreaded to make a move, lest I should be impeded by selecting the wrong diet, encasing me in a tomb of failure. Perspiration burst from every pore, and stood in cold big beads upon my forehead. The agony of suspense grew at length intolerable, and I cautiously moved forward to choose a diet, and my eyes straining from their sockets, in the hope of catching some faint ray of light to guide me in my decision-making. I proceeded for many hours; but still all was blackness and vacancy.

I breathed more freely. It seemed evident that mine was not, at least, the most hideous of fates. And now, as I still continued to move cautiously onward in trying to make a decision, there came thronging upon my recollection a thousand vague rumors of the horrors of bad diets. Of certain diets there had been strange things narrated—fables I had always deemed them—but yet strange, and too ghastly to repeat, save in a whisper. Was I left to perish of starvation in this subterranean world of darkness in dieting ignorance; or what fate, perhaps even more fearful, awaited me? That the result of non-selection would be obesity, and a fatness of more than customary bitterness, I knew too well the character of my indecision to doubt. The mode of dieting and the hour were all that occupied or distracted me.

My outstretched hands at length encountered a solid possibility. It was a plant-based diet, seemingly of colorful possibilities—some food very smooth and bright, others slimy and grotesque. I made the decision with trepidation; moving forward with all the careful distrust with which certain antique narratives had inspired me. This process, however, afforded me no means of ascertaining how quickly I could lose the desired amount of weight; as I might make several calculations, and return to the point whence I set out, without being aware of the facts; so perfectly uninformed seemed my estimates.

I therefore sought the scale which had been in my bathroom, when I first moved in; but it was gone; it had been exchanged for a cloak of ignorance. I had thought of searching the entire place in some hope of finding it in an obscure corner, so as to identify my starting weight on the same scale I would use throughout my ordeal. The difficulty, nevertheless, was but trivial; although, in the disorder of my fancy, it seemed at first insurmountable.

I tore out of my home, still in my robe and placed my trust in a navigation app to locate the nearest warehouse club store, which at length, I remembered was kitty-corner to the Walmart. In groping my way around the store, I could not fail to encounter an appropriate scale upon completing the search of each aisle. So, at least I thought: but I had not counted upon the extent of the selections, or upon my own weakness. The end aisles were full of food samples, dripping with enticements to slip up and cheat on my diet before it even began. I staggered onward for some time, when I fell to temptation. My excessive hunger induced me to remain paralyzed; and a trance soon overtook me as I gazed.

Upon stretching forth my arms, I found in my hands a humongous piece of pink frosted cookie and a bottle of soda. I was too much exhausted from my ordeal of the day to reflect upon the consequences of this circumstance, but ate and drank with enthusiasm. Shortly afterward, I resumed my tour around the warehouse, and with much toil came at last upon the area with bathroom scales.

Up to the period when I fell to temptation I had counted one hundred fifty-two paces, and upon resuming my walk, I had counted one hundred forty-eight more;—when I arrived at the scales. There were in all, then, three hundred paces; and, admitting that was quite the exercise, I presumed to have walked off the calorie equivalent of my indiscretion.

I was met, however, with many bathroom scales from which to choose, and thus I could form no guess as to the best of the lot; for I was not an expert in such things. I could not help but eeny-meeny-miny-mo-ing what was to be and upon purchasing the indiscriminate scale, returned home.

I had little object left then but to begin my plant-based diet—certainly no hope that my researches had lead me to the best diet; but a vague curiosity prompted me to continue with the one I had selected.

Quitting bad eating habits, I resolved, should begin with crossing off forbidden foods from my grocery list and immediately discarding those foods from my kitchen. At first I proceeded with extreme caution, for the plant-based diet brochure, although seemingly full of solid advice, made me feel somehow disloyal to my ooey gooey friends. At length, however, I took courage, and did not hesitate in my firm resolve; endeavoring to cross things off my list and toss food in the garbage can in as direct a way as possible. I had advanced with some ten or twelve items in this manner, when the remnant of a torn wrapper encasing my favorite dessert became entangled between my fingers. I tried flinging it off, and a piece of the delectable treat fell sadistically upon my face.

In the confusion attending my mishap, I did not immediately apprehend a somewhat startling circumstance, which yet, in a few seconds afterward, and while I still stood there contemplating my next move, arrested my attention. It was this—the sweet lump rested upon my chin, close to my lips but the upper portion of my head, although seemingly at first to have been splattered with the dessert, was untouched. At the same time my forehead seemed bathed in a clammy sweat, and the appetizing smell of the scrumptious treat arose to my nostrils. I put forward my hand, and shuddered to find that I had not moved it to wipe away my chin, but to rest at the pit of my stomach, whose emptiness, of course, I had not ascertained until this very moment, having had nothing to eat since leaving the doctor's office this morning save for the cookie and soda at the warehouse club store ... OK, and the ice cream binge too.

Groping about the kitchen for a paper towel, I succeeded in dislodging the small fragment of food, and let it fall onto the table. For many seconds I stared at the heap as it sat there, daring me to carry it to its proper place—my mouth—to relieve the hollowness I felt in my stomach. At length I took a sudden lunge for a gulp of water instead, which was succeeded by loud, gurgling noises. At the same moment there came a sound resembling the quick opening, and as rapid closing of a door—the door to ever enjoying food again. A faint gleam of light flashed suddenly through the gloom, that of my resolve to maintain a healthy weight, but it just as suddenly faded away.

The Pit and the Pendulum Diet

I saw clearly the doom which had been prepared for me, yet congratulated myself upon the timely accident by which I had escaped. Another slipup before fully engaging in a diet, and the diet would have seen me no more. And the failure just avoided, was of that very character which I had regarded as fabulously encouraging in the tales respecting diets. To the victims of such tyranny, there was the choice of minimalistic eating with its direst physical agonies of feeling starved, or gluttony with its most hideous horrors of poor health. Until now I had been resorting to the latter. By long, self-indulgent habits my health had been undone, until I trembled at the sound of my doctor's voice, and had become in every respect a fitting subject for the species of diet torture which awaited me.

Shaking in every limb, I groped my way back to continue the ceremony at my cupboards; resolving there to let tasty food perish rather than risk the terrors of failure, of which my imagination now pictured many various incarnations. In other conditions of mind I might have given into weakness and end my misery at once by a plunge into one of these scrumptious goodies; but now I took courage in my resolve. Nonetheless, I could not forget what I had read of these empty pits in the stomach—that the horror of these feelings would forever be my companion while adhering to a diet plan.

Agitation of spirit kept me awake for many long hours; but at length I again slumbered. Upon arousing before dawn, I found my way to the refrigerator. A burning thirst consumed me, and I emptied an energy drink in one gulp. I should not have procrastinated replacing the refrigerator's burnt out bulb, for in my haste I had instead drunk from a bottle of cough medicine with codeine. Scarcely had I drunk, before I became irresistibly drowsy. A deep sleep fell upon me—a sleep like that of death. How long it lasted of course, I know not; but when, once again, I unclosed my eyes, the objects around me were visible—it was daytime. By a wild sulphurous lustre, the origin of which I could not at first determine, given my drug-induced state of mind, I was enabled to see the extent of my forbidden food purge the previous night.

In its size I had been greatly mistaken. The whole of my twenty-five cubic foot refrigerator/freezer was empty. For some minutes this fact occasioned me a world of vain trouble; vain indeed! for what could be of less importance, under the terribly hungry circumstances which engulfed me, than the mere dimension of my fridge? But my soul took a wild interest in trifles, and I busied myself in endeavors to account for the error I had committed.

The truth at length flashed upon me. In my first attempt at purging unhealthy foods from my kitchen I had counted fifty-two minutes, up to the period when I encountered the torn wrapper; I must then have been distracted by the subsequent events; in fact, I had completely lost track of emptying my treasury of treats. I then slept, and upon awaking, I returned to the fridge, taking my steps in the blackness of the night—thus supposing that which was left to be much more than it actually was. My confusion in the dark prevented me from observing that I had grabbed the liquid medication and thus began my intoxicated deep sleep, which ended with what felt like a brick wall.

I had been deceived, too, in respect to the amount of items I had discarded from my cupboards. In feeling my way through them I first came to "healthy" fruit snack packages, and thus deduced an idea of great oddity; so potent is the effect of total hunger upon one arousing from an intoxicated sleep. I would make a meal out of them! The packages had a few slight depressions, or niches, at odd intervals—they had been squished behind other things for quite some time. The general shape of the packages were, nonetheless, square.

When purchased they were soft, but upon opening a package seemed now to be made of iron, or some other metal, clumped together in huge plates, whose seams or joints occasioned the depressions. The entire surface of this metallic cluster was crudely smeared in all the hideous and repulsive devices to which the eerie superstitions of marketers have given rise. The figures of fiends in aspects of menace, with skeleton forms, and other more really fearful images, overspread and disfigured the blob. I remembered buying them for Halloween trick-or-treaters—two years ago. I observed that the outlines of these monstrosities were sufficiently distinct, but that the colors seemed faded and blurred, as if from the effects of what heat had created the jumbled mess. I now noticed the floor, too, which was tile. In the centre of my being yelled the hunger from whose jaws I had not escaped; but yet would not, as the tile looked singularly as appetizing as the fruit snacks.

All this I saw indistinctly and by much effort: for my personal condition had been greatly changed during my anesthetized slumber. I now went back to the cupboards, and after an exhaustive search—now sitting on the floor—discovered a missed package of beef jerky on a lower shelf.

To my decision of starting a plant-based diet I was securely bound— or so I thought—but my resolve waned as I stared at those long strips of beef resembling belts tightening around my starving stomach. Hunger passed in many convolutions about my limbs and body, leaving at liberty only my head to contemplate my predicament, and my dominant hand to such extent that I could, by will of not much exertion, rip open the package and supply myself with food from a plastic bag which remained tightly grasped in my other hand now convulsing by my side. Hello anti-carb diet!

I saw, to my horror, that the pull strip had been removed. I say to my horror; for I was consumed with an intolerable craving. This craving, it appeared to be the design of packaging sadists to prolong: for the food in the bag was meat pungently seasoned, which could only be obtained with the aid of a sharp object.

The Pit and the Pendulum Diet

Looking upward, I assessed my surroundings trying to remember in what drawer I kept the scissors when my eyes rested upon my grandfather clock. It was some thirty or forty centimeters in width, two meters in height, and constructed much as any other. However, in one of its panels a very singular figure riveted my whole attention. It was the painted figure of Father Time as he is commonly represented, save that the bottom of his scythe appeared to continue until it morphed into the huge pendulum such as are common on these antique clocks.

There was something, however, in the appearance of this machine which caused me to regard it more attentively. While I gazed directly upward at it, I saw the fancy pendulum in motion. In an instant afterward my eyes were fixed. Its sweep was brief, and of course slow. I watched it for some minutes, somewhat in dismay, but more in wonder. Wearied at length with observing its dull movement, I turned my eyes upon another object in my home.

A slight noise attracted my notice, and, looking to the front door, I saw several enormous people traversing it. They had issued from the same gene pool as I, which lay just north of sloth. Even then, while I gazed, they came up in a group, hurriedly, with ravenous eyes, allured by the package of meat in my hand. From this it required much effort and attention to scare them to go away, though I ended up sharing most of the jerky before they did.

It might have been half the morning, perhaps even many hours, (for I took but imperfect note of time) before I was again alone and I once more cast my eyes at the pendulum. What I then saw mystified and amazed me. The sweep of the pendulum had decreased in its meter, though I had wound it tight less than a week ago, or so it seemed. I wound it once again and as a natural consequence, its velocity was much greater. But what mainly disturbed me was the idea that time had not perceptibly passed. Was dieting to be like this? Time between meals seeming to last forever?

The Pit and the Pendulum Diet

I now fantasized—with what horror it is needless to say—that the pendulum's lower extremity was formed of a crescent of glittering steel, about a foot in length from horn to horn; the horns upward, and the under edge evidently as keen as that of a razor. Like a razor also, it seemed massive and heavy, tapering from the edge into a solid and broad structure above. It was appended to a weighty rod of brass, and the whole hissed as it swung through the air, so cutting were the hunger pangs.

I could no longer doubt the doom prepared for me by the torture of time. My cognizance of hunger had become known to every fiber of my being—the hunger whose horrors had been destined for so bold a former anti-dieter as myself—the hunger, typical of one with a bottomless pit for a stomach, and regarded by me as though I had been banished to the Sahara without sustenance. The plunge into this dieting hunger I had avoided by refusing to diet my entire life, I knew that panic, or entrapment into torment, formed an important portion of all the twistedness of any diet. Having failed to diet in the past, was it part of such demonic plans to hurl me into the abyss of starvation; and thus (there being no alternative to dieting other than unhealthy fatness) a different and a milder deprivation would always await me? Milder! I half smiled in my agony as I thought of such application of such a term.

What fear does strike the heart to tell of the long, long hours of horror more than mortal, during which I counted the rushing vibrations of the steel! Inch by inch—second by second—with a cadence only appreciable at intervals that seemed ages—down and still down into the depths of despair I came! Days passed—or it might have been days for how it felt—before time swept so closely, ever so closely, to my next meal. The odor of my stinging breath forced itself into my nostrils. I prayed—I wearied heaven with my prayer for time's more speedy passing. I grew frantically mad, and struggled to force myself to think of anything but the sweep of the fearful pendulum. And then I fell suddenly calm, and smiled at the glittering metronome, as a child at some rare bauble.

The Pit and the Pendulum Diet

There was another interval of utter insensibility; it was brief; for in regard to the lapsing of time there had been no perceptible progress. But it might have been long; for I knew there were internal demons who took note of my fallibility, and who could have arrested my hunger pains at a moment's notice. Upon coming to my senses, though, I felt very—oh, inexpressibly sick and weak, as if through a long famine. Even amid the agonies of that period, the human nature craved food.

With painful effort I outstretched my left hand, insofar as my lack of will permitted, and took possession of the small remnant of jerky which had been spared me by my relatives. As I put a portion of it within my lips, there rushed to my mind a half formed thought of joy—of hope. Yet what business had I with hope? It was, as I say, a half formed thought—people have many such which are never completed. I felt that it was of joy—of hope; but felt also that it had perished in its formation. In vain I struggled to perfect—to regain it. Long suffering had nearly annihilated all my ordinary powers of mind. I was an imbecile—an idiot—I had eaten too soon.

The tempo of the pendulum was at odds with the length of time I could bear to wait. I saw that even designing to cross-my-heart-and-hope-to-diet would not, could not, provide enough strength of will. Such acute hunger would fray the fabric of my nerves—it would return and repeat its operations—again—and again.

Notwithstanding the terrifically vast amount of time still left to wait (OK, by now it was only some thirty minutes or more) and the ticking vigor of the clock, sufficient to divide asunder the strongest will of steel, and the fraying of my nerves would be all that, for several minutes, was all I could stand to wait under such circumstances. And at this thought I paused. I dared not go farther than this reflection. I dwelt upon it with a determination of attention—as if, in so dwelling, I could arrest here the pains of hunger.

The Pit and the Pendulum Diet

I forced myself to reason: I had no food left in the place to eat anyway. Upon the sound of the tick tock as time continued to pass I threw on my coat and felt a peculiar thrilling sensation as the friction of car tires against the road produced motion toward the health food store. I pondered upon all this lightheartedness until my teeth were visible through my grin.

Downtown—steadily downtown I crept—traffic was a nightmare. I took a frenzied pleasure in contrasting how long it would take to get downtown at this minimum velocity instead of at the posted speed. To the right—to the left—far and wide—nothing but a sea of cars with the occasional shriek of slammed brakes; slowly to the store I plodded ready to pounce like a tiger on my fellow drivers! I alternately laughed and howled at them as the idea of their incapability to drive properly grew predominant.

Downtown—certainly, relentlessly inching downtown! An inattentive driver swung into my lane coming to within three inches of my car! I shouted violently, furiously, shaking my left arm out the window. This was from the elbow to the wrist—I shall not recount what gesture my hand almost made. I fumbled to reach the end of my seat belt, to the buckle beside me, as my mouth continued the tirade. With great effort I stopped my hand from pressing the release button, my hand went no farther. Had I released the fastener, I would have jumped out of the car and seized that driver's throat in an attempted to arrest my frustration with this traffic—and my hunger. I might as well have attempted to arrest an avalanche!

Downtown—still unceasingly—still inevitably heading downtown! I gasped and struggled at each stop-start. I shrunk convulsively at its every recurrence. My eyes followed the exhaust from tailpipes swirling outward, then upward with the eagerness of asphyxiating mother earth and her inhabitants and I felt the most pointless despair; my eyes closed themselves spasmodically at the rising smoke, although at this point choking to death from the fumes would have been a relief, oh! how unspeakable!

Still I quivered in every nerve to think how slight the progress of this congested mass of machines would facilitate increased pollution that would keenly collect in my bosom. It was hope that prompted the nerve to quiver—the frame to shrink. It was hope—the hope that triumphs on the road—that whispers to the idling driver even in the center of the gridlock.

At last I saw that some ten or twelve feet would bring my vehicle in contact with the parking lot to the health food store, and with this observation there suddenly came over my spirit all the keen, collected calmness of despair. For the first time it now occurred to me that every parking space, or stall, which lined the lot, was occupied. I was fit to be tied.

The first stroke of luck would be catching someone leaving from one of the diagonal spaces before anyone else wanting the spot could arrive. I would need to be so detached from my emotions as to not be courteous and also not become unwound from slipping my car in before another and risking an accident. But how fearful, in that case, the proximity of the steel! The result of the slightest miscalculation how dangerous! Was it likely, moreover, that the parking lot designers had foreseen and arranged for this possibility—sadistic schemers!

Was it probable that the people leaving the store now and crossing toward the truck three spaces in front of me would provide the parking spot I so desired? Dreading to find otherwise, and, as it seemed, in last hope frustrated, I so far elevated my head as to obtain a distinct view of the situation. The seat belt enveloped my limbs and body closely in all directions as I stretched as far off the seat as I possibly could—seeing as best I could the path of the departing shoppers.

The Pit and the Pendulum Diet

Scarcely had I dropped my head back into its original position, when the truck's brake lights flashed upon my eyes. Of what I can only describe as sheer joy that no other car was in the vicinity, I quickly parked in the vacated spot.

As I entered the store I realized I did not even have half of an unformed idea as to what I should purchase. Deliverance from my hunger to which I have previously alluded, and of which a fraction of the answer to my dilemma only floated indeterminately through my brain when I thought of food relieving my burning stomach lead to the only viable conclusion I could think of. The whole thought was now present—feeble, scarcely sane, scarcely definite,—but still entire. I proceeded at once, with the nervous energy of despair, to buy one of everything.

I arrived back home at the same instant that my immediate family did. For many hours the vicinity of the kitchen table upon which I had laid bowls and platters of the food I had just purchased, had been literally swarming with my non-dieting relatives. They were wild, bold, ravenous; their red eyes glaring upon me for my healthy food choices as if they waited but for me to bring out 'the good stuff'. "To what food," I thought, "have they been accustomed?" Like I had to ask.

They had devoured, in spite of all my efforts to prevent them, all but a small remnant of the contents of the bowls of food I had placed before them. I had fallen into an habitual see-saw, or wave of the hand about the platters to slow their pace: and, at length, the unconscious uniformity of the movement deprived it of effect. In their voracity the annoying 'guests' frequently fastened their sharp fangs in my food. With the particles of the oily and spicy vittles which now remained, I thoroughly scrubbed from the dishes wherever I could yank them from their reach; then, raised my hand to signify the feeding frenzy had come to an end.

The Pit and the Pendulum Diet

At first the ravenous animals were startled and terrified at the change—at the cessation of gluttony. They shrank alarmedly back; a couple sought the exit. But this was only for a moment. I had, unfortunately, underestimated their voracity. Observing that I remained without motion, one or two of the boldest leaped for the bags of food I had not yet put away. This seemed the signal for a general rush. Forth from the bags they pulled fresh feed. They clung to the grub—they engulfed it, and devoured my hundreds of dollars' worth of groceries. The measured movement of my waving arms disturbed them not at all. Avoiding my shrieks they busied themselves with the anointed task at hand. They pressed—they swarmed upon the food leaving behind wrappers in ever accumulating heaps.

Barely perceiving my withering throat from shouting; their cold glances sought my own; I was half stifled by their thronging pressure; disgust, for which the world has no name, swelled my bosom, and chilled, with a heavy clamminess, my heart. Yet one minute, and I felt that the struggle would be over, the food vanished. Clearly I perceived the loosening of my tongue. I knew that if I spoke what I was thinking in that one instance, my relationship with these people must surely be severed. With a more than human resolution I kept still.

I had not erred in my discretion—nor had I endured in vain. I at length felt that I would be free, free from this heritage of overindulgence. The bonds of overeating now hung in shreds in my mind. The impact of this feeding frenzy already pressed upon my soul. It had divided my past from my future. It had cut through to the fibre beneath. Twice again it struck, and a sharp sense of pain shot through every nerve. But the moment of escape had arrived. At a wave of my hand my feasting family hurried senselessly away. With a steady movement—cautious, erratic, timid, and slow—I slid from the embrace of my upbringing and beyond the reach of precedent. For the moment, at least, I was free.

The Pit and the Pendulum Diet

Free!—and yet still in the grasp of my hunger! I was scarcely able to wrestle away a few morsels of food from my voracious relatives and now that they had left, I had the horrible thought to eat their dropped crumbs from off the kitchen's stone cold floor. Before I could change my mind, I quickly pulled out my old, loud vacuum and when the motion of the hellish machine ceased and I beheld how the crumbs had been drawn up, by some invisible force, through the hose to the clear dirt collection cup, it was a lesson which I took desperately to heart—get (food) while the gettin's good. I undoubtedly needed to be watchful of my every decision.

Free!—I had but escaped my upbringing in one form of agony—the bad habit of overeating—to be delivered now unto a fate worse than death in some other—an abhorrence to exercise. With that thought I rolled my eyes and nervously dressed in exercise attire hoping it would somehow hem me in from jiggling about.

Something unusual—some change which, at first, I could not appreciate distinctly—it was obvious, had taken place in the apartment. For many minutes of a dreamy and trembling abstraction, I busied myself in vain, unconnected conjecture—could I exercise without passing out?

During this period, I became aware, for the first time, of the origin of a glowing light which illumined an adjoining room—I had left the TV on. The eerie light proceeded from the crack of a barely opened door, about half an inch in width, extending up and down the door.

I entered the room and at the base of one wall appeared to my view the remote. I sat down to pick it up and wondered if I'd now be able to separate myself from the floor. Surfing through the channels, I endeavored for half an hour, but of course in vain, to look through the available exercise programs on TV for a routine that I could at least attempt to imitate. At last, I found the "King of Exercise" and decided to begin.

The Pit and the Pendulum Diet

As I arose at the attempt, the mystery of the alteration in the room broke at once upon my understanding—I had become lightheaded from my enthusiasm to stand too quickly. I observed that, although the outlines of the figures on the TV were sufficiently distinct, yet the colors seemed blurred and indefinite—was I starting to pass out?

I regained my bearings and these colors had now assumed, and were momentarily assuming, a startling and most intense brilliancy, that gave to the unnaturally thin and inhuman portrayals of exuberant exercisers an aspect that might have nauseated even firmer nerves than my own. They probably didn't even get that thin by doing *these* exercises.

Sunken eyes, of a wild and appalling cheerfulness, glared upon me from the screen as I began to mimic their movements. My untrained body moved in a thousand inaccurate directions, where it had never been before, and gleamed with the bright lustre of streaming sweat that I could not force my imagination to regard as unreal.

Unreal!—Even while I breathed there came to my nostrils the smell of a heated locker room. A suffocating odour pervaded my senses! A deeper fervor settled each moment in the eyes that glared from the television at my agonies! A richer tint of crimson diffused itself over every inch of my skin. I panted! I gasped for breath! There could be no doubt of the design of my tormentors—oh! most unrelenting! oh! most demoniac of athletes! I shrank from the glowing box in the centre of the room.

Amid the thought of my looming heat stroke, the idea of the coolness of a tall glass of sweet lemonade came over my soul like balm. I almost rushed to the deadly brink of that 300 calorie beverage. Instead I threw my straining vision back toward the TV.

The Pit and the Pendulum Diet

The glare from the screen illumined my red, blotchy hide. Yet, for a wild moment, did my spirit refuse to comprehend the meaning of what I saw. At length it forced—it wrestled its way into my soul—it burned itself in upon my shuddering reason.—Oh! for that instructor's voice to speak!—oh! horror!—oh! any horror but this! With a shriek, I rushed away from the TV, and buried my face in my hands—weeping bitterly. The voice had declared double time!

My body temperature continued to rapidly increase in spite of having paused, and once again I looked up, shuddering as with a fit of a fever. There had been a second change in the call to "feel the pain"—and now the change was obviously in the form of more difficult exercises. As before, it was in vain that I, at first, endeavoured to appreciate or understand how to perform this new set of exercises. But not long was I left in doubt as to my next move. The oppressive punishment had been hurried by my two-fold approach—excessive exercise and habitual hunger—and there was to be no more association with the "King of Terrors".

My situation had been boxlike where I had painted myself into a corner, not contemplating the possibility of thinking outside the proverbial box. I now saw that the two angles I had employed to improve my health were too intense—and I, consequently, too dense.

The fearful difference from my past perspective and what I now realized quickly increased with the low rumbling or moaning sound emanating from my belly. In an instant the apartment had shifted its form from a prison cell into that of an oasis. But the alteration stopped not there—I neither hoped nor desired it to stop. I could have clasped all the diet brochures to my bosom as a garment of eternal peace. "Balance," I said aloud, "a happy medium, a measured approach, any approach but that of the empty pit of my stomach!" Fool I might have remained while knowing that heat stroke was my destiny due to the compelling expectations that urged me on.

The Pit and the Pendulum Diet

Could I resist the societal norms thrust upon me? or, if even that, could I withstand peer pressure? And now, fatter and fatter grew my resolve—and hopefully not my midsection—with a rapidity that left me no time for contemplation. Its enemy, of course, its greatest menace, would come to me over and over again with each new day. I would shrink back from the pressures of the world every now and again—but the insight I had now gained would press me resistlessly onward. At length for my once seared and writhing mind, there was no longer an inch of foothold by those archaic societal body images that used to imprison me. I struggled no more, but the agony of my soul found vent in one loud, long, and final scream of release. I felt that I had tottered upon the brink—but I had overcome! I would no longer avert my eyes from any mirror--

There will always be a discordant hum of human voices! There will be, at times, a loud blast as of many trumpets or a harsh grating as of a thousand thunders! The 'ideal' body images will continue to burn into my consciousness, but I will fight back! Do I still need to lose weight? Yes. Will I kill myself doing it? No! I need to be health-conscious and not an extremist.

There will be outstretched arms to catch my own as I start to fall or faint from my efforts. They will keep me from sinking into despair. They will come from the general public as well as from rational friends. The French fry shall continue to pass my lips as I shout 'Holy Toledo' in delight at its savor ... but less occasionally.

Ridicule at the hands of my enemies has lost its sting.

www.ingramcontent.com/pod-product-compliance
Lightning Source LLC
Chambersburg PA
CBHW062034280526
45787CB00005B/2317